Autism Diet for Children

Beginner's Guide and Cookbook for Autism

Table of Contents

Introduction

Introduction

Parents often encounter problems when it comes to feeding autistic children. Kids with autism will typically start to pick one kind of food over the other or will have varying preferences every day.

While doctors and nutritionists cannot clearly point out the reason for certain autistic behavior, parents can still manage to feed their children with nutritious foods to optimize their development.

Most children with autism can benefit from alternative diets in addition to conventional therapy. Some parents with autistic children claim that eliminating certain foods from their children's diet reduces the symptoms of the condition.

Doctors suggest choosing types of food that are similar to what the child normally eats. Take it slowly when you are trying to introduce new foods. Remember that many children are resistant to change.

You should also consider following certain diets to ensure that your child gets all the vitamins and nutrients needed. Gluten-free, grain-free, dairy-free and processed sugar free diets can be beneficial for children with autism.

As soon as your child gets used to the food, reward them with something that they like. It does not have to be material in nature. A warm hug can already serve as a positive reinforcement for them.

Chapter 1 – Why are Gluten-free, Grain-free, Dairy-free and Processed Sugar-free Diet Plans Effective in Treating ADHD?

Gluten- free, grain- free, dairy- free and processed sugar- free diets have been getting a lot of attention in the autism community because many studies show that children with ADHD showed dramatic improvements in their speech and behavior by removing these substances from their diet.

According to studies, autistic children have abnormal response to gluten, grain, dairy and sugar than other normal and healthy children their age. Some theories also propose that people with autism cannot properly digest gluten and dairy which can worsen their symptoms and cause several health problems.

A research study in New Jersey found that autistic children have more antibodies that react to gluten which can lead to intestinal abnormalities.

Children with autism process peptides and protein differently from other people which can also trigger negative reactions. The brain is said to treat protein like opiate and chemicals and leads the child to act in a different way.

Removing foods that contain gluten, grain, processed sugar and dairy from the diet plans of autistic children is effective in reducing and improving their cognitive behavior and speech. These diet plans aim to eliminate the source of discomfort in most autistic children and improve their intestinal health.

Gluten-free, grain-free, processed sugar-free and dairy-free diet plans are also effective in treating autism because these promote proper absorption of nutrients from the foods they eat.

Supplying autistic children with the right nutrients is valuable in improving their overall health and their mental and emotional development. This diet can also improve their behavior and mood.

Chapter 2 - Gluten-free and Grain-free Diet for ADHD Sufferers / Autistic Children

Autism is a developmental disorder that can affect a child's ability to communicate and interact with other people. Studies show that alternative diet treatments can help reduce the symptoms.

Gluten is a protein that is found in some grains. A lot of products in the market contain gluten. Gluten is often used as a binding agent for most baked goods.

Gluten-free and grain-free diet plans encourage the elimination of gluten found in wheat, rye and barley. While it could be quite difficult to avoid all types of food that contain gluten, parents can still exert some effort in controlling their child's gluten consumption.

Gluten-free diet became popular as a treatment for celiac disease. It is also known to help people lose weight. Gluten-free diet is one of the most effective alternative treatments for autistic children.

History of Gluten Consumption

Humans have been consuming gluten for centuries but technological advances have changed the way food is being processed. Most grains purchased today contain more gluten because of the selective breeding implemented by most farms.

Overuse of antibiotic can also affect the balance of bacteria in the gut, making it a lot difficult to manage gluten. Also, the hyper-sanitized environment can weaken the immune system and trigger different kinds of sensitivities.

Effects of Gluten to Autistic Children

One of the main reasons why parents are advised not to feed their autistic children with foods that are rich in gluten and grain is that these substances can cause the immune system to react negatively.

Gluten can damage the intestinal walls and cause symptoms like stomach pain and vomiting. Gluten-free and grain-free diet proponents even say that most children with autism encounter gastrointestinal difficulties, making it more difficult for them to properly digest grains and gluten-rich products.

This problem can greatly affect autistic children in different ways. One negative effect is that it can result to high gluteomorphines (protein by-products) level in the body. These protein by-products can drastically affect the behavior of autistic children.

These by-products may reduce the desire of children to interact socially while also blocking their pain messages and increasing their confusion. The problem is that children with autism may not be able to properly communicate these symptoms and they can have more temper tantrums to express their discomfort.

Removing gluten and grain from their diet is an effective treatment for autism because this can reduce the level of protein by-products in their body, which is a major help in improving their mood and behavior.

When you decide on gluten free diet, most bread and grain products will be eliminated. Therefore, make sure that your child still gets enough vitamins, fiber and minerals.

Fortunately, more and more food companies are accommodating special diets due to the number of people suffering from gluten sensitivity.

You can also consult your doctor and a dietician to help tailor a good diet for your child.

Why is Gluten-free and Grain-free Diet Effective for Autistic Children?

- **Prevents gastrointestinal problems**

A study proposes that children with autism may not be able to digest gluten properly and as a result, it acts like opiates in the body. It can alter the child's behavior, response and perceptions to his surroundings.

Some scientists even detected a significant amount of protein peptides in the urine of autistic children. Gluten prevents the intestinal walls from absorbing nutrients which can lead to malnutrition.

It also increases stomach problems like bloating, gas and abdominal cramps. Removing gluten and grain from the diet of autistic children enables them to digest protein better.

- **Lessens headache and brain fog**

Children with autism often experience headache, brain fog and depression after eating foods with gluten. This effect may be attributed to a molecule called cytokine which is released when gluten is ingested.

Cytokines has also been linked to the development of Alzheimer's, Parkinson's and Autism.

- **Reduces skin and body inflammation**

Gluten causes inflammation in body tissues. People with autism may also experience joint pain and muscle cramps, as well as numb limbs because of eating gluten.

Skin inflammation can also occur and skin rashes may appear. Children with autism often see improvement in skin inflammation several days after switching to a gluten-free diet.

- **Increases energy and improves mood**

Children with autism may exhibit low energy levels. Since gluten can cause slight malnutrition, it can also trigger a drop in energy levels and leave your children feeling exhausted.

People with gluten intolerance may report an overall feeling of weakness.

Caution:

Gluten-free and grain-free advocates say that even a small amount of gluten, dairy or wheat can have a negative impact to the behavior and health of a child with autism. As a parent, you have to make sure that you avoid letting your child accidentally eat the wrong foods.

You can avoid this by reading the labels of certain food products carefully before including them in the diet of your child. Note that gluten, dairy and wheat are usually hidden ingredients in packed goods, so you have to do your research and read the labels.

Informing the teachers, therapists and other important adults in the life of your autistic child that you are starting to feed him/her with grain-free and gluten-free foods is also essential. This is to ensure that your child won't eat the wrong foods when you are not around.

Chapter 3 – Dairy-free and Processed Sugar-free Diet for Autistic Children

Scientific studies have shown that many autistic children experience better temperament when they are on a dairy and sugar-free diet.

While medical professionals are still debating on the relationship of dairy and autistic symptoms, some of them theorize that dairy can cause gastrointestinal problems and thus worsen the child's behavior.

Dairy and sugar-free diet is also one of the most popular specialized diets for autistic children. The reason behind the popularity of these diet plans is that these are useful in reducing autistic symptoms in children including impulsive behaviors, speech problems and lack of focus.

Advocates of these diet plans also say that autistic children often react poorly to foods that are rich in processed sugar, dairy and gluten, so eliminating these substances from the diet of your autistic child makes a lot of sense.

A diet which is free of processed sugar and dairy is also useful for your child especially if he is also suffering from allergies and bowel issues. While this type of diet requires you to eliminate a lot of foods from the meals of your child, he can still enjoy a variety of vegetables, meat and fruits.

It is possible to replace dairy products with substitutes such as coconut, rice, soy and nuts. With your creativity and some experimentation, finding the foods that your autistic child will enjoy while also fitting in his diet is possible.

Benefits of Dairy-free Diet for Autistic Children

- **Decreases the risk of skin inflammation**

Doctors suggest eliminating dairy and processed sugar from the diet of autistic children because these can be flushed out of the system faster. Most autistic children get clearer skin after eliminating dairy products from their diet.

Many people are not aware that they are allergic to dairy which can cause skin inflammation. Other studies also suggest that milk contains hormones that can aggravate acne.

- **Prevents sensitivity reactions**

Allergic reactions to traditional milk are prevalent in young children with autism. The severity of milk allergy can range from life threatening conditions like anaphylaxis to mild symptoms like hives. Eliminating dairy can effectively prevent any sensitivity reaction to lactose.

- **Avoids food allergies**

Among the significant factors that contribute in the development of autism symptoms are food chemicals that reach the brain because of ineffective absorption and digestion.

Few years after birth, humans may lose the ability to digest milk and naturally lose lactase which is an enzyme that helps digest lactose in milk.

Many autistic children are also lactose intolerant which means that they are not able to digest dairy products effectively. Autistic children that are also suffering from food intolerances and allergies can benefit from the diet because it promotes healthier digestion and reduces allergic reactions.

- **Reduces exposure to antibiotics and hormones**

Large quantities of antibiotics are given to cows to prevent infection. These antibiotics can be passed to their milk. The consumption of cow's milk can increase the levels of insulin like growth hormone.

It can also increase the risk of colon, lung and breast cancer for autistic children since they usually have weaker immune system due to the large dose of medication they are prescribed with.

Sugar-free Diet

Sugar is one of the most popular ingredients in the world. It is usually added to baked goods, coffee and confectionaries. Sugar also comes in different varieties with some of them claiming to be better than the others.

Sugar, especially the processed type, is considered as an empty food since it does not give the body the nutrient that it needs. Sugar has also been linked to major diseases like heart disease, cancer and hyperactivity in children with autism. Chewing unprocessed sugar cane can provide the body with vitamins and minerals.

However, once it goes through industrial processing, all the nutrients from the sugar cane are removed and all that is left is the sweet taste and substances that are difficult to digest.

One of the most dangerous effects is when acid accumulates in the brain and interferes with cell development. The cells begin to die once it does not have enough oxygen. This can result to a delay in your child's brain development.

The body can also refuse to digest the sugar and store it in the liver. This is transformed into fatty acids that can cloud major organs such as the heart and kidneys.

Children with autism usually have food allergies and intolerance. This can result in damaged intestines and unbalanced bacterial environment.

Children with autism can also experience ear infection because of the overuse of antibiotics. Continuous use of antibiotic can easily lead to yeast overgrowth. The presence of sugar in the body only worsens the condition since yeast thrives on sugar.

Yeast also produces toxins including a chemical called alcohol. The chemical is carried in the brain where it can inhibit brain development.

This leads to irritability, sugar craving, depression, reduced motor skills and a decrease in attention span.

Benefits of Processed Sugar-free diet to Autistic Children

- **Reduction of headache and fatigue**

Sugar consumption is often linked to energy fluctuation. Children with autism usually feel bloated and lethargic after consuming foods that are rich in sugar. Eliminating sugar from your child's diet can help maintain a good energy level throughout the day.

- **Less mood swings**

Autistic children are known to have unexpected mood swings. Keeping sugar levels in check can help maintain enough levels of serotonin, a chemical that can affect moods.

Low serotonin levels can lead to insomnia, fatigue and anxiety and worsen your child's behavior.

The main problem with sugar is that it is converted into energy quickly and once it is gone, the body experiences energy crash. Once their serotonin level is controlled, ADHD and autism patients usually feel better physically and emotionally.

- **Weight loss benefit**

A significant percentage of autistic children have obesity and weight problems. Sugar can easily be stored as fat. Completely eliminating sugar can lead to dramatic weight loss for the first two weeks.

Encouraging physical activity along with a processed sugar-free diet can help them lose weight faster. You can still incorporate healthy sugar from fruits and vegetables and experience the same weight loss benefits.

- **Overall health**

Sugar is very damaging to the body. Eliminating it can easily prevent disease, cancer, obesity and mental problems, most especially for children with autism.

To conclude, parents must consider removing dairy, grain, processed sugar and gluten from the diet of their autistic children. Doing this is effective in reducing the symptoms of autism while also showing great improvements in the eye contact, mood and digestive health of your affected child.

Note that dairy-free and sugar-free diet plans may not only benefit children with autism; these can also benefit everyone in the family.

Many families who initially switched to specialized diets to help their children with autism gradually started to incorporate it to their lifestyle as well.

Breakfast Ideas

Lox and Avocado Crêpes

Prep Time: 10 minutes

Dehydrating Time: 7 - 10 hours

Servings: 2

INGREDIENTS

4 - 6 oz smoked salmon

1 ripe avocado

1/2 lemon

1 sprig fresh dill

1 teaspoon sesame seeds (black or white)

Crêpes

1 young coconut (plus coconut water)

1/3 cup raw sunflower seeds

1/2 cup flax seeds

1/2 white ground pepper (or 1/4 teaspoon ground black pepper)

1/2 teaspoon Celtic sea salt

Water

INSTRUCTIONS

1. For *Crêpes*, add flax to food processor or high-speed blender. Process until finely ground, up to 5 minutes. Add sunflower seeds and process until finely ground, about 1 minute.

2. Remove flesh and water from young coconut. Add to processor with salt and pepper. Process until smooth batter forms, about 1 - 2 minutes. Add enough water to reach desired consistency.

3. Place parchment paper or dehydrator sheets on dehydrator trays.

4. Spread batter on prepared sheets. Place trays in dehydrator and set to 115 degrees F for 6 - 8 hours.

5. Remove trays from dehydrator. Remove *Crêpes* from parchment or dehydrator liners, flip, and place directly on dehydrator tray. Place trays back in dehydrator and continue dehydrating 1 - 2 hours, until surface is dry but *Crêpe* is still pliable.

6. Remove from dehydrator and cut into desired shape and size. Set aside.

7. Finely chop fresh dill. Cut avocado in half and remove pit. Slice flesh in peel.

8. Lay *Crêpes* flat and top with line of smoked salmon down center. Scoop portion of sliced avocado over smoked salmon. Sprinkle on chopped dill. Roll up *Crêpes* and transfer to serving dish.

9. Top *Crêpes* with squeeze of lemon juice and sprinkle on sesame seeds. Serve immediately.

Turkey Jerky Bacon

Prep Time: 10 minutes*

Dehydrating Time: 4 - 8 hours

Servings: 4

INGREDIENTS

4 oz organic turkey (dark meat)

2 tablespoons coconut aminos (or liquid aminos)

2 tablespoons tamari (or liquid aminos or coconut aminos)

1 tablespoon lemon juice (or raw apple cider vinegar)

1 tablespoons Celtic sea salt

1/2 teaspoon garlic powder

1/2 teaspoon onion powder

1/2 teaspoon smoked paprika

Pinch cayenne pepper

INSTRUCTIONS

1. Prepare two sheet parchment. Lay one on cutting board.
2. Cut turkey into 1/4 inch strips and lay in single layer on parchment. Pound with tenderizing side of kitchen mallet. Cover turkey with second parchment sheet, then pound with flat side of tenderizing mallet to 1/8 inch thickness.
3. *Place turkey strips in medium mixing bowl or shallow dish. Add coconut aminos, tamari, lemon juice, salt and spices. Mix well to coat. Cover and place in refrigerator for 8 hours, or overnight.

4. Remove turkey from refrigerator and lay in single layer on dehydrator trays. Place trays in dehydrator and set to 120 degrees F for 4 - 8 hours.

5. After 4 hours dehydrating time, remove trays from dehydrator and test turkey by bending. If it cracks, remove and serve immediately. Or store in airtight container.

6. If still flexible, place back in dehydrator and continue dehydrating up to 4 hours, or until desired texture is achieved.

Stone-wrought Coop

Prep time: 5 minutes

Cook time: 3-6 minutes

INGREDIENTS

2 cage-free eggs

1 small onion

1 clove garlic

½ red bell pepper

1 tbsp extra virgin olive oil

¼ tsp smoked paprika

¼ tsp ground black pepper

INSTRUCTIONS

1. Finely chop onion, garlic and red bell pepper.
2. Pour extra virgin olive oil into a pan over medium heat.
3. Crack eggs and pour into a small bowl. Combine with onion, garlic and red bell pepper and whisk until mixed together.
4. Pour contents of bowl into pan and add smoked paprika and ground black pepper. Scramble until desired doneness. Serve.

Ancient Egg Muffins

Prep time: 5 minutes

Cook time: 15-20 minutes

INGREDIENTS

1 tbsp olive oil

1 tbsp coconut oil

6 cage-free eggs

1 onion

½ yellow bell pepper

½ red bell pepper

¼ tsp ground black pepper

¼ tsp Celtic sea salt

INSTRUCTIONS

1. Preheat oven to 350. Whisk all 6 eggs in a bowl. Chop the onion and bell pepper into small pieces.

2. In a pan, combine olive oil with onion over medium-high heat for 2 minutes. Add peppers and cook another 2 minutes.

3. Remove onion/peppers from heat and let cool a few minutes. Combine them with the eggs. Add the Celtic sea salt and ground black pepper and mix.

4. Coat a muffin pan with the coconut oil. Fill each muffin cup with the egg/pepper/onion mix. Do not fill a muffin cup more than ¾ full.

5. Place the pan in the oven and bake 10-15 minutes, removing the pan from the oven when the tops of the muffins get fluffy and golden brown.

6. Remove the muffins from the pan and serve.

Sizzled Chicken Wraps

Prep time: 5 minutes

Cook time: 3 minutes

INGREDIENTS

4 slices of chicken deli meat

1 tbsp olive oil

1 small onion

1 red bell pepper

1 avocado

¼ tsp garlic powder

INSTRUCTIONS

1. Remove the nut from the avocado and mash it into a paste. Chop the pepper and onion into small pieces.
2. Combine the garlic powder, pepper and onion in the bowl with the avocado and mix well.
3. Add the olive oil in a pan over low heat and heat the chicken mildly, turning frequently, for 3 minutes.
4. Remove the chicken from heat and place ¼ of the avocado/pepper/onion mixture onto each piece.
5. Wrap the chicken up into tubes and serve.

Green Monster Kale and Poached Eggs

Prep time: 10 minutes

Cook time: 12 minutes

INGREDIENTS

1 handful kale

2 cage-free eggs

1 small onion

1 clove garlic

1 tbsp extra virgin olive oil

¼ tsp ground black pepper

1 tsp low-sodium horseradish (optional)

INSTRUCTIONS

1. Chop the onion and mince the garlic. De-stem and wash the kale. Leaving a bit of water on the kale is ideal.

2. In a saucepan, add 1 tbsp extra virgin olive oil over medium heat. Add onion and cook until it begins to lose its opaqueness, about 5 minutes.

3. Add kale to saucepan and cover until kale is soft and green, about 5 minutes. Add garlic and stir, then cook another 2 minutes and remove from heat.

4. Fill a saucepan half full of water. Bring the water to a boil, then reduce heat below a boil and hold it there.

5. One by one, crack the eggs into a small cup or bowl and, with the lip of the cup or bowl close to the water's surface, dump the egg

into the water. If necessary, nudge the eggwhites closer to the yolks to keep them together.

6. Once all the eggs are in the water, remove the pan from heat and cover it. Let sit for 4 minutes until all eggs are cooked, then remove eggs from pan.

7. Place the greens on a plate and the two eggs on top of the greens. Top with horseradish if desired. Serve.

Lunch Ideas

Mexican Tomato Soup

Prep Time: 35 minutes

Servings: 2

INGREDIENTS

Shrimp

10 - 12 large shrimp

1 - 1 1/2 cups lemon juice (about 8 lemons)

1/2 jalapeño pepper

Gazpacho

2 cups tomato juice (about 4 large tomatoes)

2 plum tomatoes

1/2 red bell pepper

1/2 red onion

1/2 cucumber

Small bunch fresh cilantro

2 garlic cloves

2 tablespoons raw apple cider vinegar(optional)

2 tablespoons raw oil (coconut, walnut, almond, sesame, etc.) (optional)

1 teaspoon ground black pepper

1 teaspoon Celtic sea salt

INSTRUCTIONS

1. For *Shrimp*, Peel, devein and remove tails from shrimp. Mince jalapeño and juice lemons. Add to small bowl and mix. Shrimp should be completely covered in lemon juice. Place in refrigerator for 30 minutes, or until shrimp are opaque.

2. For Gazpacho, juice large tomatoes in juicer. Or add to food processor or high-speed blender and process, then strain into medium mixing bowl.

3. Peel cucumber and seed. Seed plum tomatoes. Seed, stem and vein bell peppers. Peel onion and garlic. Dice veggies and onion, and mince garlic. Add to tomato juice.

4. Add salt, pepper, vinegar and oil (optional). Mix well, then place in refrigerator.

5. Chop cilantro and set aside.

6. Remove shrimp from refrigerator and drain lemon juice and jalapeños. Rinse if desired.

7. Mix shrimp into tomato mixture. Pour into serving bowls and top with chopped cilantro. Serve chilled.

Texas Chili

Prep Time: 10 minutes*

Servings: 2

INGREDIENTS

5 - 6 plum tomatoes

1/2 teaspoon dried cumin

1/4 teaspoon chili powder

1/4 teaspoon onion powder

1/4 teaspoon garlic powder

1 teaspoon fresh oregano leaves (or 1/4 teaspoon dried oregano)

1/2 teaspoon ground black pepper

1/4 teaspoon cayenne pepper or red pepper flakes (optional)

1 teaspoon Celtic sea salt

1 teaspoon chia seed (or flax seed)

1/2 cup raw cashews

Water

INSTRUCTIONS

1. *Soak raw cashews in enough water to cover overnight in refrigerator. Drain and rinse. Set aside.
2. Grind chia or flax in food processor or high-speed blender. Set aside.
3. Juice tomatoes. Or add to food processor or high-speed blender and process. Add enough water to reach desired consistency, if necessary. Then strain.

4. Add tomato juice, ground chia or flax, 1/2 of soaked cashews, salt, pepper and spices to blender. Process until smooth, about 1 - 2 minutes.
5. Stir in remaining soaked cashews.
6. Pour into serving bowls and serve immediately.

Creamy "Cheese" and Broccoli Soup

Prep Time: 10 minutes*

Servings: 2

INGREDIENTS

1 1/2 - 2 cups broccoli florets

1 red bell pepper

1 garlic clove

1/4 cup raw oil (coconut, walnut, almond, sesame, etc.)

1 cup nutritional yeast

1 tablespoon coconut aminos (or tamari)

1 tablespoon onion powder

1/2 teaspoon Celtic sea salt

1/4 teaspoon ground white pepper (or ground black pepper)

2 cups raw cashews

Water

INSTRUCTIONS

1. * Soak raw cashews in enough water to cover at least 2 hours, or overnight in refrigerator. Drain and rinse. Set aside.
2. Chop broccoli florets into pieces and set aside.
3. Seed and vein bell pepper. Peel garlic. Add to food processor or high-speed blender with soaked cashews, nutritional yeast, coconut aminos, salt, pepper and enough water to process until smooth, about 2 - 3 minutes.
4. Pour into serving bowl and top with broccoli. Serve immediately.

Caesar Salad

Prep Time: 10 minutes

Servings: 1

INGREDIENTS

2 cups chopped romaine lettuce

Almond Parmesan

1/4 cup raw almonds

1 teaspoon raw apple cider vinegar

1 teaspoon nutritional yeast (optional)

1/4 teaspoon garlic powder

1/4 teaspoon onion powder

1/4 teaspoon dried oregano

1/4 teaspoon Celtic sea salt

Raw Caesar Dressing

2 tablespoons raw cashews (or raw sunflower seeds)

2 tablespoons raw sunflower seeds

1 tablespoon raw pine nuts (or raw sesame seeds or raw tahini)

2 tablespoons lemon juice

1 garlic clove

3/4 teaspoon coconut aminos (or nutritional yeast)

1/2 teaspoon dried dill (optional)

Cracked or ground black pepper, to taste

Water

INSTRUCTIONS

1. Rinse, dry and plate romaine lettuce.

2. For *Almond Parmesan*, add almonds, vinegar, salt, spices and nutritional yeast (optional) to food processor or high-speed blender. Process until almonds are coarsely ground and resemble ground parmesan cheese. Set aside.

3. For *Raw Caesar Dressing*, peel garlic and add to food processor or high-speed blender with lemon juice. Process until smooth. Then add remaining ingredients and process until smooth, about 1 - 2 minutes. Add enough water to reach desired consistency.

4. Drizzle *Raw Caesar Dressing* over salad and sprinkle with *Almond Parmesan*. Serve immediately.

Smoked Salmon Avocado Salad

Prep Time: 10 minutes

Servings: 1

INGREDIENTS

Salad

2 cups soft lettuce leaves (looseleaf or butterhead varieties)

1/2 cup watercress or dandelion leaves (optional)

2 oz smoked salmon

1/2 avocado

1 sprig fresh dill

1 tablespoon caviar (optional)

Avocado Cream Dressing

1/2 avocado

1 sprig fresh dill

1 tablespoon lemon juice

1/2 teaspoon ground black pepper

1/2 tcaspoon Celtic sea salt

1/2 coconut

Water

INSTRUCTIONS

1. For *Salad*, rinse, dry and plate lettuce and watercress or dandelion leaves (optional). Cut avocado in half and remover pit. Dice or slice avocado flesh in peel, then scoop onto greens. Lay smoked salmon over greens.

2. For *Avocado Cream Dressing*, remove coconut flesh from peel and add to food processor or high-speed blender with enough water to reach desired consistency. Process until smooth and creamy, about 1 - 2 minutes. Strain mixture through nut milk bag and place back into blender.

3. Scoop remaining avocado flesh into blender. Add lemon juice, 1 sprig dill, salt and pepper and process until well combined and smooth, about 1 minute.

4. Drizzle *Avocado Cream Dressing* over salad. Mince remaining dill and sprinkle over salad. Dollop caviar over salad (optional).

5. Serve immediately.

Pesto Tomato Caprese

Prep Time: 5 minutes

Servings: 2

INGREDIENTS

1 large yellow tomato

1 large red tomato

Small bunch fresh basil

Celtic sea salt, to taste

Crack or ground black pepper, to taste

Basil Pesto

2 cups basil leaves (packed)

1/4 cup raw pine nuts

1/2 - 1/3 cup raw oil (coconut, walnut, almond, sesame, etc.)

2 garlic cloves

1/2 lemon (or 1 tablespoon raw apple cider vinegar)

1/4 teaspoon Celtic sea salt

INSTRUCTIONS

1. For *Basil Pesto*, peel garlic and add to food processor or high-speed blender with squeeze of 1/2 lemon. Process until finely chopped. Add pine nuts, basil, oil and salt and process until finely ground, about 1 minute.

2. Slice tomatoes and plate in alternating colors. Sprinkle with salt and pepper. Chiffon basil leaves.

3. Spread *Basil Pesto* over tomato slices and top with fresh basil. Serve immediately.

Cilantro Taco Salad

Prep Time: 10 minutes

Servings: 1

INGREDIENTS

Salad

2 cups lettuce (chopped)

1/2 cup cilantro (chopped)

1 plum tomato

1/2 small onion

1 garlic clove

1 avocado

1/2 lime

1/2 jalapeño

Paprika, to taste

Ground black pepper, to taste

Celtic sea salt, to taste

Raw Taco Meat

1/4 cup walnuts

2 - 3 sundried tomatoes

1/4 teaspoon cumin

1/8 teaspoon garlic powder

1/8 teaspoon smoked paprika

1/8 teaspoon ground white pepper (or ground black pepper)

1/8 teaspoon teaspoon Celtic sea salt

INSTRUCTIONS

1. For *Salad*, rinse, dry and plate lettuce and cilantro. Reserve pinch of cilantro in small mixing bowl.

2. Peel onion and dice. Reserve 1/2 of onion in separate mixing bowl and add remaining onion to reserved cilantro. Remove seeds from jalapeño ad mince. Dice tomato. Add to onion and cilantro with squeeze of lime. Sprinkle on pinch of salt and pepper, and mix to combine. Set aside.

3. Cut avocado in half and remove pit. Scoop flesh into bowl with reserved onion. Peel garlic and mince, and add to avocado with squeeze of lime. Sprinkle on salt, pepper and paprika to taste. Mash slightly and mix with fork until well combine but still chunky. Set aside.

4. For *Raw Taco Meat*, add walnuts, sundried tomatoes, salt, pepper and spices to food processor or high-speed blender. Pulse until coarsely ground.

5. Top *Salad* with *Raw Taco Meat*, avocado and tomato mix. Serve immediately.

Asian Shrimp Lettuce Wraps

Prep Time: 35 minutes

Servings: 2

INGREDIENTS

4 large lettuce leaves (thin, flexible ribs)

1 cup cabbage (shredded)

1 small carrot

1/2 green onion

1/2 inch piece fresh ginger

1 small garlic clove

1/2 teaspoon raw sesame seeds

1/2 teaspoon coconut aminos (or tamari or raw apple cider vinegar)

1 teaspoon raw oil (sesame, coconut, walnut, almond, etc.)

Shrimp

10 - 12 medium shrimp

3/4 cup lemon juice (about 5 lemons)

1 teaspoon red pepper flakes

1/2 green onion (scallion)

Almond Sauce

2 tablespoons raw oil (sesame, coconut, walnut, almond, etc.)

1/4 cup raw almond butter (or 1/2 cup raw almonds)

1 tablespoon lemon juice (or coconut aminos or tamari)

1/2 small mild chili pepper

Water

INSTRUCTIONS

1. For *Shrimp*, slice green onion and reserve half in small mixing bowl. Peel, devein and remove tails from shrimp. Add to separate bowl with lemon juice, remaining green onion and red pepper. Mix to combine. Shrimp should be completely covered in lemon juice. Place in refrigerator for 30 minutes, or until shrimp are opaque.

2. Peel ginger and garlic, and finely grate or mince. Add to green onion with coconut aminos and oil. Mix to combine. Set aside.

3. For *Almond Sauce*, add oil, almond butter or almonds, lemon juice and chili pepper to food processor or high-speed blender. Process until smooth and creamy, about 1 - 2 minutes. Add enough water to reach desired consistency. Transfer to serving dish.

4. Shred cabbage and carrot and add to ginger mixture. Toss to coat.

5. Rinse, dry and plate lettuce leaves. Drain shrimp and layer onto lettuce. Top with cabbage mixture and sprinkle on sesame seeds. Roll up lettuce wraps and serve with *Almond Sauce*.

Chicken Fries with Garlic Aioli

Prep Time: 10 minutes

Cook Time: 15 minutes

Servings: 2

INGREDIENTS

8 oz boneless, skinless chicken breast

1 egg

1/2 cup almond meal

1 teaspoon flax meal (or ground chia seed)

1 teaspoon ground black pepper

1/2 teaspoon paprika

1/2 teaspoon onion powder

1/2 teaspoon garlic powder

1/2 teaspoon chili powder

1/2 teaspoon sea salt

Garlic Aioli

1/2 - 3/4 cup coconut oil

1 egg yolk

2 garlic cloves

1/2 small lemon

1/4 teaspoon ground white pepper (or black pepper)

1/4 teaspoon sea salt

3 tablespoons flavorful oil (black truffle, walnut, almond, sesame, etc.) (optional)

INSTRUCTIONS

1. Heat large pan over medium-high heat and coat with coconut oil.

2. For *Garlic Aioli*, peel garlic and add to food processor or blender with egg yolk, juice of 1/2 lemon, salt and pepper. Process until smooth, scraping down sides of vessel.

3. While processor or blender is running, very slowly drizzle in enough coconut oil to create thick mayo-like mixture. Drizzle in flavorful oil as well will processor runs (optional). If mixture is runny, drizzle in more coconut oil while processor runs until thickened. Pour into serving dish and refrigerate.

4. Slice chicken into half width-wise, creating twice the fillets. Try to slice at thickest portion to keep all fillets equal thickness.

5. Slice chicken fillets into long, 1/2 inch wide strips. Place strips between two paper towels and press to absorb excess moisture.

6. In a shallow dish, blend almond meal, flax or chia meal, spices and salt.

7. Beat egg in small mixing bowl. Toss chicken strips in beaten egg to lightly coat, then dredge in seasoned almond meal.

8. Carefully place coated chicken strips into hot oil and fry about 2 - 3 minutes, until golden brown and cooked through. Turn with tongs half way through cooking.

9. Drain cooked chicken on paper towel, then transfer to serving dish.

10. Serve hot with *Garlic Aioli*.

Quick Chili

Prep Time: 5 minutes

Cook Time: 20 minutes

Servings: 4

INGREDIENTS

1 lb lean grass-fed ground beef (or elk, bison, turkey or chicken)

15 oz (1 can) organic tomato sauce

6 oz (1 can) organic tomato paste

1 small onion

1 bell pepper

2 cloves garlic

2 tablespoons chili powder

1 tablespoon ground cumin

1 tablespoon smoked paprika (or paprika)

1 teaspoon Mexican oregano (or dried oregano)

1 teaspoon ground black pepper

1 teaspoon sea salt

1/2 teaspoon cayenne pepper

1 tablespoon coconut oil

sea salt, to taste

INSTRUCTIONS

1. Heat medium pot over medium-high heat. Add 1 tablespoon coconut oil.

2. Peel onion and garlic. Stem and seed bell pepper. Chop and add to food processor or bullet blender. Pulse until finely minced.

3. Add to skillet and sauté for about 1 minute. Add ground beef and spices. Brown beef for about 5 minutes. Stir with whisk to break up meat well, or wooden spoon to keep beef chunkier.

4. Add whole cans of tomato sauce and paste. Stir to combine.

5. Bring to a simmer, then reduce heat to medium and cover loosely with lid to prevent splatter. Simmer about 10 minutes. Stir occasionally.

6. Use large serving spoon or ladle to serve hot.

Dinner Ideas

Zucchini Pasta with Sundried Tomato Sauce

Prep Time: 5 minutes

Servings: 2

INGREDIENTS

1 large zucchini

Zesty Tomato Sauce

2 medium tomatoes (or 3 plum tomatoes)

5 sundried tomatoes

2 tablespoons raw cashews (or 1 tablespoon raw cashew butter)

2 large garlic cloves

Small bunch fresh basil leaves

1 small fresh oregano sprig

Ground black pepper, to taste

Cayenne pepper, to taste

Celtic sea salt, to taste

INSTRUCTIONS

1. Carefully slice zucchini with spiralizer, vegetable peeler, or sharp knife. Sprinkle with pinch of salt, pepper and cayenne. Gently toss to coat and set aside.

2. For *Zesty Tomato Sauce*, remove basil and oregano leaves from stems. Peel garlic. Add to food processor or high-speed blender with tomatoes, sundried tomatoes, cashews or cashew butter, salt, pepper and cayenne. Process until smooth, about 1 - 2 minutes.

3. Transfer zucchini pasta to serving dishes. Top with *Zesty Tomato Sauce* and serve immediately.

Zucchini Pasta with Pesto

Prep Time: 10 minutes

Servings: 2

INGREDIENTS

1 small zucchini

1 bell pepper (or 1 carrot)

Pine Nut Pesto

2 1/2 cups fresh basil leaves

1/2 cup raw pine nuts

1 garlic clove

2 tablespoons raw oil (walnut, almond, coconut, sesame, etc.)

1/4 teaspoon ground white pepper (or ground black pepper)

1/4 teaspoon Celtic sea salt

INSTRUCTIONS

1. Carefully slice zucchini with spiralizer, vegetable peeler, or sharp knife. Carefully slice carrot with spiralizer, vegetable peeler, or grater, if using. Or remove stem, seeds and veins from bell pepper, then julienne (cut into long thin slices). Set aside.

2. For *Pine Nut Pesto*, peel garlic and add to food processor or high-speed blender with basil, 2 tablespoons pine nuts, oil, salt and pepper. Process until thick, smooth mixture forms, about 1 - 2 minutes.

3. Add *Pine Nut Pesto* to veggie pasta and toss to coat. Transfer to serving dish and top with remaining pine nuts. Serve immediately.

Zucchini Fettuccini Alfredo

Prep Time: 10 minutes

Servings: 2

INGREDIENTS

1 medium zucchini

1 carrot (or 1 small sweet potato)

Alfredo Sauce

1 cup raw cashews

1 teaspoon lemon juice (or raw apple cider vinegar)

2 garlic cloves

1/2 teaspoon dried thyme

1/2 teaspoon Celtic sea salt

Water

Walnut Parmesan

1/2 cup raw walnuts

3 tablespoons nutritional yeast

1/4 teaspoon ground white pepper (or ground black pepper)

1/2 teaspoon Celtic sea salt

INSTRUCTIONS

1. Carefully slice zucchini and carrot or sweet potato with spiralizer, vegetable peeler, or grater. Set aside.
2. For *Alfredo Sauce*, peel garlic and add to food processor or high-speed blender with cashews, lemon juice, thyme and salt. Process

until smooth mixture forms, up to 5 minutes. Add enough water to reach desired consistency. Set aside.

3. For *Walnut Parmesan*, add walnuts to clean food processor or high-speed blender and process until finely ground. Add nutritional yeast, salt and pepper. Process until coarsely ground and mixture resembling parmesan cheese forms.

4. Add *Alfredo Sauce* to veggie pasta and toss to coat. Transfer to serving dish and top with *Walnut Parmesan*. Serve immediately.

Cashew Crunch Kelp Noodle Salad

Prep Time: 10 minutes*

Servings: 2

INGREDIENTS

1 package (12 oz) kelp noodles

1/2 lemon

1/2 small red bell pepper

Cashew Sauce

1 cup raw cashews

1/2 small red bell pepper

1/2 lemon

1 tablespoon coconut aminos (or raw apple cider vinegar)

2 large basil leaves

1/2 teaspoon smoked paprika

1/2 teaspoon ground black pepper

1/2 teaspoon Celtic sea salt

1/4 teaspoon ground turmeric (optional)

1/4 teaspoon smoked chili powder (optional)

Water

INSTRUCTIONS

1. *Soak 3/4 cup cashews in enough water to cover at least 4 hours, or overnight in refrigerator. Drain and rinse.

2. Drain and rinse kelp noodles. Add to medium bowl with warm water and juice of 1/2 lemon. Set aside 5 minutes.

3. Cut bell pepper in half. Remove stem, seeds and veins and set half of pepper aside. Julienne (thinly slice) remaining bell pepper and add to medium mixing bowl.

5. For *Crunchy Cashew Sauce*, add soaked cashews, bell pepper, juice of 1/2 lemon, coconut aminos, basil, salt and spices to food processor or high-speed blender. Process until smooth, about 2 minutes. Add enough water to reach desired consistency. Set aside.

4. Drain kelp noodles and add to sliced bell pepper. Add *Cashew Sauce* and toss to coat. Transfer noodles to serving dishes.

5. Roughly chop remaining 1/4 cup cashews. Sprinkle noodles and serve immediately. Or refrigerate for 20 minutes and serve chilled.

Raw Walnuts Tacos

Prep Time: 35 minutes

Servings: 2

INGREDIENTS

4 large lettuce leaves (thin, flexible ribs)

1 plum tomato

1/4 red onion (or white or yellow onion)

Medium bunch cilantro

1 avocado

1/2 lime

Taco Meat

1 cup raw walnuts

1/2 cup sundried tomatoes

1/2 teaspoon ground cumin

1/4 teaspoon garlic powder

1/4 teaspoon smoked chili powder

1/4 teaspoon Celtic sea salt

Cayenne pepper, to taste

Cashew Sour Cream

1/2 cup raw cashews

1 lemon

1/8 teaspoon Celtic sea salt

3 tablespoons cup water

1/3 cup ice

INSTRUCTIONS

6. *Soak sundried tomatoes in enough water to cover at least 2 hours, or overnight in refrigerator. Drain.

7. For *Taco Meat*, add soaked tomatoes, walnuts, salt and spices to food processor or high-speed blender. Process until chunky mixture forms, about 1 minute. Set aside

8. For *Cashew Sour Cream*, add cashews, lemon juice, salt, water and ice to clean food processor or high-speed blender. Process until smooth, about 2 minutes.

9. Chop cilantro. Dice tomato. Thinly slice onion. Cut avocado in half, then remove pit and slice in peel.

10. Fill lettuce leaves with *Taco Meat*. Scoop avocado slices onto *Taco Meat*. Drizzle on *Cashew Sour Cream*. Top with diced onion and tomato, and sprinkle of chopped cilantro. Top with squeeze of lime.

11. Fold lettuce around filling and transfer to serving dish. Serve immediately.

Tilapia Lettuce Wraps

Prep Time: 35 minutes

Servings: 2

INGREDIENTS

1 lb boneless, skinless tilapia fillets (or other white fish)

1 1/4 cup lemon juice (about 8 lemons)

4 large lettuce leaves (thin, flexible ribs)

1 cup cabbage (shredded)

1 small carrot

1/2 green onion (scallion)

Cilantro Sauce

1/2 cup raw cashews

1 lemon

1/2 inch piece fresh ginger

1 small garlic clove

Medium bunch cilantro

1/4 teaspoon Celtic sea salt

3 tablespoons water

1/3 cup ice

INSTRUCTIONS

1. Juice lemons into medium mixing bowl. Cut tilapia into 1 inch strips. Add to lemon juice and toss to coat. Tilapia should be completely covered in lemon juice. Place in refrigerator for 30 minutes, or until tilapia is opaque.

2. Carefully slice carrot with spiralizer, vegetable peeler, or grater. Shred cabbage. Slice green onion. Set aside.

3. For *Cilantro Sauce*, remove cilantro leaves form stems. Peel ginger and garlic. Add to food processor or high-speed blender with cashews, lemon juice, salt, water and ice. Process until smooth, about 2 minutes.

4. Remove tilapia from refrigerator and drain. Gently rinse, if preferred. Fill lettuce leaves with tilapia. Add shredded cabbage and carrot. Drizzle on *Cilantro Sauce*. Top with sliced green onions.

5. Fold lettuce around filling and transfer to serving dish. Serve immediately.

City Clam Chowder

Prep Time: 35 minutes

Servings: 2

INGREDIENTS

2 dozen live littleneck clams

1 - 1 1/2 cups lemon juice (about 8 lemons)

2 cups tomato juice (about 4 large tomatoes)

2 plum tomatoes

1 celery stalk

1 carrot

1 red bell pepper

1 green bell pepper

1/4 teaspoon cayenne pepper

1/2 teaspoon onion powder

1 teaspoon dried oregano

1 teaspoon dried basil

1 teaspoon ground black pepper

1 teaspoon Celtic sea salt

INSTRUCTIONS

5. Have fishmonger shuck clams. Or carefully shuck clams yourself. Reserve clam juice.

6. Juice lemons into medium mixing bowl. Add clams and toss to coat. Clams should be completely covered in lemon juice. Place in refrigerator for 30 minutes, or until clams are opaque.

7. Juice large tomatoes in juicer then add to food processor or high-speed blender. Or add to food processor or high-speed blender and process, then strain and return to processor.

8. Remove stems, seeds and veins from bell peppers. Cut red and green bell pepper in half. Cut carrot and celery stalks in half. Add half of each veggie to tomato juice with salt and spices. Process until smooth, about 2 minutes. Add to medium mixing bowl. Set aside.

9. Dice plum tomatoes, and remaining celery, carrot, and bell pepper. Add to tomato purée with reserved clam juice, salt and spices.

10. Remove clams from refrigerator and drain lemon juice. Gently rinse, if desired. Add to bowl and mix to combine.

11. Transfer to serving dish and serve immediately.

Creamy French Onion Soup

Prep Time: 15 minutes*

Dehydrating Time: 6 hours

Servings: 2

INGREDIENTS

3 cups raw almond milk (or 1 cup raw almonds + 4 cups water)

1/2 lemon

1/4 cup tamari (or coconut aminos or raw apple cider vinegar)

1 tablespoon coconut aminos (or tamari or raw apple cider vinegar)

2 tablespoons raw oil or butter (ghee, cacao butter, coconut butter, almond oil, walnut oil, coconut oil, etc.)

1/2 teaspoon dried thyme

1/2 teaspoon cracked black pepper (or ground black pepper)

Caramelized Onions

2 onions

1 tablespoon raw honey (or 2 dried pitted dates)

1 tablespoon tamari (or coconut aminos or raw apple cider vinegar)

1 tablespoon raw oil (almond, walnut, coconut, etc.)

1/4 teaspoon Celtic sea salt

INSTRUCTIONS

1. *Soak almonds in 1 cup water at least 6 hours, or overnight in refrigerator. Drain and pop off skins, if preferred.

2. For *Caramelized Onions*, add dates, tamari, oil and salt to food processor or high-speed blender and process until smooth. Add water to reach desired consistency, if necessary.

3. Or add honey, tamari, oil and salt to large mixing bowl and mix to combine. Peel onions and thinly slice. Add to bowl and toss to coat.

4. Prepare several dehydrator or parchment sheets and line dehydrator tray. Spread coated onion on prepared trays and place in dehydrator on 110 degrees F for 6 hours.

5. Add soaked almonds to high-speed blender with 3 cups water. Process until well blended and almost smooth, about 1- 2 minutes.

6. Strain mixture through nut milk bag, cheesecloth or strainer back into processor. Reserve almond pulp and dehydrate for almond flour.

7. Add juice of 1/2 lemon, coconut aminos, tamari, oil, thyme and black pepper to almond milk. Add half of *Caramelized Onions* and process until smooth, about 1 minute.

8. Add half of remaining *Caramelized Onions* and pulse until onions are roughly chopped.

9. Transfer to serving dish and top with remaining *Caramelized Onions*. Serve immediately.

Salmon Tartar Stack

Prep Time: 10 minutes*

Servings: 2

INGREDIENTS

8 oz boneless, skinless salmon fillet (sushi grade)

2 limes

1 avocado

1 shallot

1 tablespoon raw oil (coconut, walnut, almond, sesame, etc.)

1 teaspoon mustard seeds (or ground mustard)

Medium sprig fresh dill

Celtic sea salt, to taste

Ground black pepper, to taste

2 teaspoons caviar (optional)

INSTRUCTIONS

1. Have fishmonger prepare salmon fillets. Or fillet salmon and remove pin bones and skin.

2. Dice salmon and transfer to serving dish. Top with squeeze of 1/2 lime and sprinkle of salt and pepper. Place in mold to form, if preferred.

3. Peel and thinly slice shallot, then add to small mixing bowl. Juice whole lime into food processor or high-speed blender. Add oil, mustard seeds and pinch of salt and pepper. Process to combine, then add to shallots.

4. Or add lime juice, oil, ground mustard, salt and pepper to shallots. Mix to combine and set aside.
5. Cut avocado in half and remove pit. Dice flesh in peel and scoop into separate mixing bowl. Finely chop dill and add to avocado with squeeze of remaining 1/2 lime, salt and pepper. Mix to combine.
6. Add avocado dill mixture to salmon. Then top with shallot mixture and caviar (optional). Serve immediately.
7. *Or refrigerate 2 hours and serve chilled.

Simple Steak Tartar

Prep Time: 10 minutes*

Servings: 2

INGREDIENTS

10 oz beef tenderloin

Small bunch fresh parsley

1/2 lemon

2 cage-free egg yolk (optional)

2 tablespoons raw oil (coconut, walnut, almond, sesame, etc.)

1 teaspoon ground mustard (or mustard seeds)

1 shallot

1/4 teaspoon chili flakes (optional)

Ground black pepper, to taste

Celtic sea salt, to taste

INSTRUCTIONS

1. Finely dice tenderloin and parsley. Add to bowl with squeeze of lemon and pinch of salt and pepper. Mix to combine.

2. Transfer to serving dish. Place in ring mold to form, if preferred. Set aside.

3. Peel shallot and mince. Add to small mixing bowl with egg yolks (optional), mustard, oil, salt and spices. Whisk to emulsify.

4. Top tenderloin with mixture and serve immediately. Or refrigerate 20 minutes and serve chilled.

Macadamia Crusted Ahi Tuna

Prep Time: 5 minutes

Cook Time: 1 minute

Servings: 1

INGREDIENTS

8 oz ahi tuna fillet

1/4 teaspoon coconut oil

1/4 teaspoon dried thyme

1/4 teaspoon dried tarragon (optional)

1/4 cup whole macadamia nuts (shelled)

1 small garlic clove teaspoon

1 small shallot teaspoon

1/2 teaspoon ground white pepper (or black pepper)

1/2 teaspoon sea salt

2 tablespoons coconut oil

INSTRUCTIONS

1. Heat medium pan over medium-high heat. Add 2 tablespoons coconut oil to pan.

2. Chop macadamia nuts well. Peel and finely mince garlic and shallot. Set aside.

3. Rub top and bottom of fillet with 1/4 teaspoon coconut oil, salt, pepper, thyme and tarragon (optional).

4. Press 1/2 chopped macadamia nuts into each side of fillet.

5. Add garlic and shallots to hot oiled pan and sauté for just a second. Do not burn.

6. Carefully place fish in pan and sear 15 - 30 seconds on each side, for rare to medium rare. Carefully flip half way through cooking.
7. Transfer fillet to serving dish and serve hot with mixed greens or favorite veggies.

Parchment Baked Salmon

Prep Time: 5 minutes

Cook Time: 20 minutes

Servings: 1

INGREDIENTS

8 oz salmon fillet (deboned, skin-on)

6 - 8 medium asparagus stalks

1/2 lemon

1 basil sprig

1 rosemary sprig

1 teaspoon coconut oil

Pinch black pepper

Pinch sea salt

Parchment paper

Kitchen twine

INSTRUCTIONS

1. Place large sheet pan on bottom rack of oven. Preheat oven to 400 degrees F. prepare parchment sheet.

2. Place salmon in middle of parchment sheet skin-side down and sprinkle with salt and pepper. Place asparagus stalks next to salmon. Cut lemon into thin slices and place over fish and asparagus. Rub herbs between palms, then lay basil and rosemary sprig over lemon slices. Drizzle 1 teaspoon coconut oil over salmon and asparagus.

3. Gather edges of parchment up over salmon and tie tightly with kitchen twine to form sealed pouch.

4. Place pouch directly on hot baking sheet in hot oven. Bake for 20 minutes.

5. Remove from oven and carefully transfer pouch to serving plate. Carefully open pouch to release steam.

6. Serve hot.

Snack Ideas

Sausage And Peppers

Prep Time: 5 minutes

Cook Time: 10 minutes

Servings: 4

INGREDIENTS

4 Italian sausage links (pork, chicken, etc.)

1 white onion

1 bell pepper

INSTRUCTIONS

1. Heat large skillet over medium heat. Add 1 tablespoon coconut oil.
2. Peel onion. Stem and seed pepper. Roughly chop onion and pepper. Slice sausage into 3/4 inch slices.
3. Add sausage to hot oiled skillet and sauté about 2 minutes. Then add onion and peppers. Sauté about 8 minutes, until sausage is cooked through and browned.
4. Serve hot.

Spicy Chicken Bites

Prep Time: 5 minutes

Cook Time: 10 minutes

Servings: 4

INGREDIENTS

8 oz boneless skinless chicken

1/2 cup almond meal

1 teaspoon flax meal

1 teaspoon paprika

1/2 teaspoon cayenne pepper

1/2 teaspoon red pepper flakes

1/2 teaspoon ground black pepper

1/2 teaspoon sea salt

1 egg

1 jalapeño pepper

2 garlic cloves

2 oz organic spicy brown mustard

Coconut oil (for cooking)

INSTRUCTIONS

1. Heat a medium skillet over medium high heat. Lightly coat pan with coconut oil.

2. Slice chicken into 1x1 inch strips. Arrange slices between 2 sheets of parchment and pound with kitchen mallet or rolling pin to flatten slightly. Place flattened pieces between two paper towels to absorb excess moisture.

3. In a shallow dish, blend almond meal, flax meal, dry spices and salt.

4. Add egg , jalapeño and peeled garlic to food processor or bullet blender. Process until fairly smooth. Pour into shallow dish.

5. Dip chicken pieces into jalapeño egg, then dredge in seasoned almond meal.

6. Carefully place coated chicken pieces into hot oil and fry about 2 minutes, until golden brown and cooked through. Turn with tongs half way through.

7. Drain cooked chicken on paper towel, then transfer to serving dish.

8. Serve hot with spicy mustard.

Simple Guacamole

Prep Time: 5 minutes

Cook Time: 5 minutes

Servings: 4

INGREDIENTS

2 avocados

1 shallot

1 small tomato

1 bunch cilantro

Half lime

2 teaspoons paprika

1/2 teaspoon ground cumin

1/2 teaspoon ground black pepper

1/2 teaspoon sea salt

INSTRUCTIONS

1. Peel and finely dice shallot. Dice tomato and cilantro. Add to small mixing bowl.
2. Slice avocados in half, pit, and scoop flesh into bowl. Add 1 teaspoon paprika, 1/2 teaspoon cumin, 1/2 teaspoon black pepper and 1/2 teaspoon salt.
3. Mash avocado and mix ingredients well with fork. Transfer to serving dish and squeeze on juice of half a lime. Sprinkle with remaining teaspoon of paprika.
4. Serve immediately. Or refrigerate 30 minutes, and serve chilled.

Green Deviled Eggs 'N Ham

Prep Time: 5 minutes

Cook Time: 10 minutes

Servings: 4

INGREDIENTS

8 eggs

1 avocado

1/2 teaspoon ground black pepper

1/2 teaspoon salt

2 oz natural ham

2 tablespoons fresh dill

INSTRUCTIONS

1. Bring medium pot of lightly salted water to boil. Gently add eggs to hot water with tongs and cook about 8 - 10 minutes.
2. Drain eggs in colander and cool in cold water.
3. Crack shells and peel eggs. Cut eggs in half lengthwise and scoop out yolks into small bowl. Arrange whites on platter with center hollows facing up.
4. Mash avocado, salt and pepper with egg yolks until smooth. Dice ham and dill, separately.
5. Scoop avocado blend into each egg white hollow and sprinkle with ham, then dill.
6. Refrigerate about 20 minutes. Serve chilled.

Pigs In A Blanket

Prep Time: 20 minutes

Cook Time: 15 minutes

Servings: 4

INGREDIENTS

1 package(26 count) nitrate-free/nitrite-free mini hot dogs

3 egg whites

1/4 cup almond flour

1/4 cup coconut flour

1 tablespoon cold coconut oil

1/2 teaspoon baking powder

Pinch garlic powder

Pinch sea salt

2 oz organic mustard

INSTRUCTIONS

1. In separate medium bowl, mix almond and coconut flours with baking powder. Cut-in cold coconut oil, then add pinch of garlic powder and salt. Mixture should be crumbly. Refrigerate 15 - 20 minutes.
2. Preheat oven to 400 degrees F. Line sheet pan with parchment or lightly coat with coconut oil.
3. Whisk egg whites in medium bowl until white and frothy, just before soft peaks develop.
4. Gently fold egg whites into refrigerated flour mixture until just combined.

5. Flatten 1 level teaspoon of dough into a rectangle in your fingers. Place one sausage in middle of dough wrap it around the sausage. Repeat with remaining sausage and dough.
6. Place wrapped sausages on prepared sheet pan and bake about 15 minutes, until dough is golden brown and links are heated through.
7. Serve hot with mustard.